I0421665

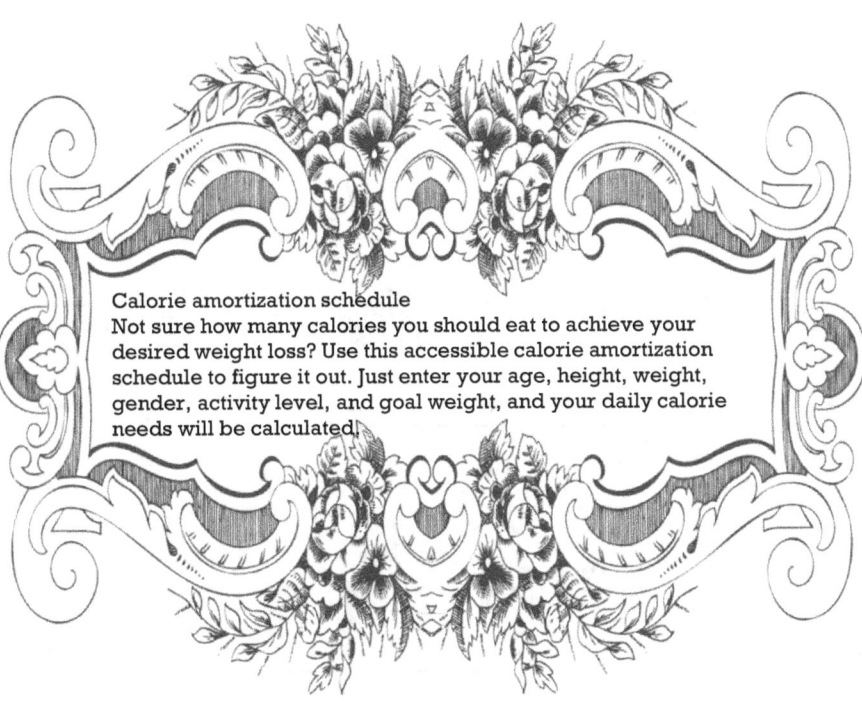

Calorie amortization schedule
Not sure how many calories you should eat to achieve your desired weight loss? Use this accessible calorie amortization schedule to figure it out. Just enter your age, height, weight, gender, activity level, and goal weight, and your daily calorie needs will be calculated.

CALORIES AMORTIZATION SCHEDULE

Extra Active	Exercise 6-7 Days/Week + Physical Job/2x Training
I Want my Weight to	
Decrease	

Goal Start Date ....../...../2........			Goal Target Date ....../...../2........		
Date	Week Day		Weight	BMR	Cal Consumed
....		....	....	....	....
....		....	....	....	....
....		....	....	....	....
....		....	....	....	....
....		....	....	....	....
....		....	....	....	....
....		....	....	....	....

It's not recommended that you decrease your calorie intake by more than 1000 calories below your daily calorie needs or consume less than 1800 calories per day.

Goal target date is based on the recommended average weight loss of .45 kg per week.

Measurement System		Current Weight		Age	
Height in m	Centimeters	Goal Weight		Gender	
Initial Daily Calorie Needs		Initial Daily Calorie Intake		Calories to Burn	
Cal Burned	Cal Deficit	Cal Remaining	Kgs Remaining	Loss	% of Goal

CALORIES AMORTIZATION SCHEDULE

Extra Active	Exercise 6-7 Days/Week + Physical Job/2x Training
I Want my Weight to	
Decrease	

Goal Start Date ....../...../2........			Goal Target Date ....../...../2........		
Date	Week	Day	Weight	BMR	Cal Consumed
....		....	....	....	....
....		....	....	....	....
....		....	....	....	....
....		....	....	....	....
....		....	....	....	....
....		....	....	....	....
....		....	....	....	....

It's not recommended that you decrease your calorie intake by more than 1000 calories below your daily calorie needs or consume less than 1800 calories per day.

Goal target date is based on the recommended average weight loss of .45 kg per week.

Measurement System		Current Weight		Age	
Height in m	Centimeters	Goal Weight		Gender	
Initial Daily Calorie Needs		Initial Daily Calorie Intake		Calories to Burn	
Cal Burned	Cal Deficit	Cal Remaining	Kgs Remaining	Loss	% of Goal

CALORIES AMORTIZATION SCHEDULE

Extra Active	Exercise 6-7 Days/Week + Physical Job/2x Training
I Want my Weight to	
Decrease	

Goal Start Date ....../...../2........			Goal Target Date ....../...../2........		
Date	Week Day		Weight	BMR	Cal Consumed
....		....	....	....	....
....		....	....	....	....
....		....	....	....	....
....		....	....	....	....
....		....	....	....	....
....		....	....	....	....
....		....	....	....	....

It's not recommended that you decrease your calorie intake by more than 1000 calories below your daily calorie needs or consume less than 1800 calories per day.

Goal target date is based on the recommended average weight loss of .45 kg per week.

Measurement System		Current Weight		Age	
Height in m	Centimeters	Goal Weight		Gender	
Initial Daily Calorie Needs		Initial Daily Calorie Intake		Calories to Burn	
Cal Burned	Cal Deficit	Cal Remaining	Kgs Remaining	Loss	% of Goal

CALORIES AMORTIZATION SCHEDULE

Extra Active	Exercise 6-7 Days/Week + Physical Job/2x Training
I Want my Weight to	
Decrease	

Goal Start Date ....../...../2........	Goal Target Date ....../...../2........

Date	Week Day	Weight	BMR	Cal Consumed
....	....	....	....	....
....	....	....	....	....
....	....	....	....	....
....	....	....	....	....
....	....	....	....	....
....	....	....	....	....
....	....	....	....	....

It's not recommended that you decrease your calorie intake by more than 1000 calories below your daily calorie needs or consume less than 1800 calories per day.

Goal target date is based on the recommended average weight loss of .45 kg per week.

Measurement System		Current Weight		Age	
Height in m	Centimeters	Goal Weight		Gender	
Initial Daily Calorie Needs		Initial Daily Calorie Intake		Calories to Burn	
Cal Burned	Cal Deficit	Cal Remaining	Kgs Remaining	Loss	% of Goal

CALORIES AMORTIZATION SCHEDULE

Extra Active	Exercise 6-7 Days/Week + Physical Job/2x Training
I Want my Weight to	
Decrease	

Goal Start Date ....../...../2........			Goal Target Date ....../...../2........		
Date	Week Day		Weight	BMR	Cal Consumed
....		....	....	....	....
....		....	....	....	....
....		....	....	....	....
....		....	....	....	....
....		....	....	....	....
....		....	....	....	....
....		....	....	....	....

It's not recommended that you decrease your calorie intake by more than 1000 calories below your daily calorie needs or consume less than 1800 calories per day.

Goal target date is based on the recommended average weight loss of .45 kg per week.

Measurement System		Current Weight		Age	
Height in m	Centimeters	Goal Weight		Gender	
Initial Daily Calorie Needs		Initial Daily Calorie Intake		Calories to Burn	

Cal Burned	Cal Deficit	Cal Remaining	Kgs Remaining	Loss	% of Goal

CALORIES AMORTIZATION SCHEDULE

Extra Active	Exercise 6-7 Days/Week + Physical Job/2x Training
I Want my Weight to	
Decrease	

Goal Start Date ....../...../2........	Goal Target Date ....../...../2........

Date	Week Day	Weight	BMR	Cal Consumed
....	....	....	....	....
....	....	....	....	....
....	....	....	....	....
....	....	....	....	....
....	....	....	....	....
....	....	....	....	....
....	....	....	....	....

It's not recommended that you decrease your calorie intake by more than 1000 calories below your daily calorie needs or consume less than 1800 calories per day.

Goal target date is based on the recommended average weight loss of .45 kg per week.

Measurement System		Current Weight		Age	
Height in m	Centimeters	Goal Weight		Gender	
Initial Daily Calorie Needs		Initial Daily Calorie Intake		Calories to Burn	
Cal Burned	Cal Deficit	Cal Remaining	Kgs Remaining	Loss	% of Goal

CALORIES AMORTIZATION SCHEDULE

Extra Active	Exercise 6-7 Days/Week + Physical Job/2x Training
I Want my Weight to	
Decrease	

Goal Start Date			Goal Target Date		
....../...../2........			....../...../2........		

Date	Week Day	Weight	BMR	Cal Consumed
....	....	....	....	....
....	....	....	....	....
....	....	....	....	....
....	....	....	....	....
....	....	....	....	....
....	....	....	....	....
....	....	....	....	....

It's not recommended that you decrease your calorie intake by more than 1000 calories below your daily calorie needs or consume less than 1800 calories per day.

Goal target date is based on the recommended average weight loss of .45 kg per week.

Measurement System	Current Weight		Age	

Height in m	Centimeters	Goal Weight		Gender	

Initial Daily Calorie Needs	Initial Daily Calorie Intake		Calories to Burn	

Cal Burned	Cal Deficit	Cal Remaining	Kgs Remaining	Loss	% of Goal

CALORIES AMORTIZATION SCHEDULE

Extra Active	Exercise 6-7 Days/Week + Physical Job/2x Training
I Want my Weight to	
Decrease	

Goal Start Date	Goal Target Date
....../...../2........	....../...../2........

Date	Week Day	Weight	BMR	Cal Consumed
....	....	....	....	....
....	....	....	....	....
....	....	....	....	....
....	....	....	....	....
....	....	....	....	....
....	....	....	....	....
....	....	....	....	....

It's not recommended that you decrease your calorie intake by more than 1000 calories below your daily calorie needs or consume less than 1800 calories per day.

Goal target date is based on the recommended average weight loss of .45 kg per week.

Measurement System		Current Weight		Age	
Height in m	Centimeters	Goal Weight		Gender	
Initial Daily Calorie Needs		Initial Daily Calorie Intake		Calories to Burn	

Cal Burned	Cal Deficit	Cal Remaining	Kgs Remaining	Loss	% of Goal

CALORIES AMORTIZATION SCHEDULE

Extra Active	Exercise 6-7 Days/Week + Physical Job/2x Training			
I Want my Weight to				
Decrease				
Goal Start Date ....../...../2........		Goal Target Date ....../...../2........		
Date	Week Day	Weight	BMR	Cal Consumed
....	....	....	....	....
....	....	....	....	....
....	....	....	....	....
....	....	....	....	....
....	....	....	....	....
....	....	....	....	....
....	....	....	....	....

It's not recommended that you decrease your calorie intake by more than 1000 calories below your daily calorie needs or consume less than 1800 calories per day.

Goal target date is based on the recommended average weight loss of .45 kg per week.

Measurement System		Current Weight		Age	
Height in m	Centimeters	Goal Weight		Gender	
Initial Daily Calorie Needs		Initial Daily Calorie Intake		Calories to Burn	

Cal Burned	Cal Deficit	Cal Remaining	Kgs Remaining	Loss	% of Goal

CALORIES AMORTIZATION SCHEDULE

Extra Active	Exercise 6-7 Days/Week + Physical Job/2x Training
I Want my Weight to	
Decrease	

Goal Start Date	Goal Target Date
....../...../2........	....../...../2........

Date	Week Day	Weight	BMR	Cal Consumed
....	....	....	....	....
....	....	....	....	....
....	....	....	....	....
....	....	....	....	....
....	....	....	....	....
....	....	....	....	....
....	....	....	....	....

It's not recommended that you decrease your calorie intake by more than 1000 calories below your daily calorie needs or consume less than 1800 calories per day.

Goal target date is based on the recommended average weight loss of .45 kg per week.

Measurement System		Current Weight		Age	
Height in m	Centimeters	Goal Weight		Gender	
Initial Daily Calorie Needs		Initial Daily Calorie Intake		Calories to Burn	
Cal Burned	Cal Deficit	Cal Remaining	Kgs Remaining	Loss	% of Goal

CALORIES AMORTIZATION SCHEDULE

Extra Active	Exercise 6-7 Days/Week + Physical Job/2x Training			
I Want my Weight to				
Decrease				

Goal Start Date			Goal Target Date		
....../...../2........			....../...../2........		

Date	Week Day		Weight	BMR	Cal Consumed
....		....	....	....	....
....		....	....	....	....
....		....	....	....	....
....		....	....	....	....
....		....	....	....	....
....		....	....	....	....
....		....	....	....	....

It's not recommended that you decrease your calorie intake by more than 1000 calories below your daily calorie needs or consume less than 1800 calories per day.

Goal target date is based on the recommended average weight loss of .45 kg per week.

Measurement System		Current Weight		Age		
Height in m	Centimeters	Goal Weight		Gender		
Initial Daily Calorie Needs		Initial Daily Calorie Intake		Calories to Burn		
Cal Burned	Cal Deficit	Cal Remaining	Kgs Remaining	Loss		% of Goal

CALORIES AMORTIZATION SCHEDULE

Extra Active	Exercise 6-7 Days/Week + Physical Job/2x Training
I Want my Weight to	
Decrease	

Goal Start Date	Goal Target Date
...../...../2........	...../...../2........

Date	Week	Day	Weight	BMR	Cal Consumed
....		....	....	....	....
....		....	....	....	....
....		....	....	....	....
....		....	....	....	....
....		....	....	....	....
....		....	....	....	....
....		....	....	....	....

It's not recommended that you decrease your calorie intake by more than 1000 calories below your daily calorie needs or consume less than 1800 calories per day.

Goal target date is based on the recommended average weight loss of .45 kg per week.

Measurement System	Current Weight		Age	

Height in m	Centimeters	Goal Weight		Gender	

Initial Daily Calorie Needs	Initial Daily Calorie Intake	Calories to Burn	

Cal Burned	Cal Deficit	Cal Remaining	Kgs Remaining	Loss	% of Goal

CALORIES AMORTIZATION SCHEDULE

Extra Active	Exercise 6-7 Days/Week + Physical Job/2x Training
I Want my Weight to	
Decrease	

Goal Start Date ....../...../2........	Goal Target Date ....../...../2........

Date	Week Day	Weight	BMR	Cal Consumed
....	....	....	....	....
....	....	....	....	....
....	....	....	....	....
....	....	....	....	....
....	....	....	....	....
....	....	....	....	....
....	....	....	....	....

It's not recommended that you decrease your calorie intake by more than 1000 calories below your daily calorie needs or consume less than 1800 calories per day.

Goal target date is based on the recommended average weight loss of .45 kg per week.

Measurement System	Current Weight		Age	

Height in m	Centimeters	Goal Weight		Gender	

Initial Daily Calorie Needs	Initial Daily Calorie Intake		Calories to Burn	

Cal Burned	Cal Deficit	Cal Remaining	Kgs Remaining	Loss	% of Goal

CALORIES AMORTIZATION SCHEDULE

Extra Active	Exercise 6-7 Days/Week + Physical Job/2x Training
I Want my Weight to	
Decrease	

Goal Start Date			Goal Target Date		
....../...../2........			....../...../2........		

Date	Week Day	Weight	BMR	Cal Consumed
....	....	....	....	....
....	....	....	....	....
....	....	....	....	....
....	....	....	....	....
....	....	....	....	....
....	....	....	....	....
....	....	....	....	....

It's not recommended that you decrease your calorie intake by more than 1000 calories below your daily calorie needs or consume less than 1800 calories per day.

Goal target date is based on the recommended average weight loss of .45 kg per week.

Measurement System	Current Weight		Age	

Height in m	Centimeters	Goal Weight		Gender	

Initial Daily Calorie Needs	Initial Daily Calorie Intake		Calories to Burn	

Cal Burned	Cal Deficit	Cal Remaining	Kgs Remaining	Loss	% of Goal

CALORIES AMORTIZATION SCHEDULE

Extra Active	Exercise 6-7 Days/Week + Physical Job/2x Training				
I Want my Weight to					
Decrease					

Goal Start Date ....../...../2........			Goal Target Date ....../...../2........		
Date	Week Day		Weight	BMR	Cal Consumed
....		....	....	....	....
....		....	....	....	....
....		....	....	....	....
....		....	....	....	....
....		....	....	....	....
....		....	....	....	....
....		....	....	....	....

It's not recommended that you decrease your calorie intake by more than 1000 calories below your daily calorie needs or consume less than 1800 calories per day.

Goal target date is based on the recommended average weight loss of .45 kg per week.

Measurement System		Current Weight		Age	
Height in m	Centimeters	Goal Weight		Gender	
Initial Daily Calorie Needs		Initial Daily Calorie Intake		Calories to Burn	
Cal Burned	Cal Deficit	Cal Remaining	Kgs Remaining	Loss	% of Goal

CALORIES AMORTIZATION SCHEDULE

Extra Active	Exercise 6-7 Days/Week + Physical Job/2x Training
I Want my Weight to	
Decrease	

Goal Start Date ....../...../2........			Goal Target Date ....../...../2........		
Date	Week Day		Weight	BMR	Cal Consumed
....		....	....	....	....
....		....	....	....	....
....		....	....	....	....
....		....	....	....	....
....		....	....	....	....
....		....	....	....	....
....		....	....	....	....

It's not recommended that you decrease your calorie intake by more than 1000 calories below your daily calorie needs or consume less than 1800 calories per day.

Goal target date is based on the recommended average weight loss of .45 kg per week.

Measurement System		Current Weight		Age	
Height in m	Centimeters	Goal Weight		Gender	
Initial Daily Calorie Needs		Initial Daily Calorie Intake		Calories to Burn	
Cal Burned	Cal Deficit	Cal Remaining	Kgs Remaining	Loss	% of Goal

CALORIES AMORTIZATION SCHEDULE

Extra Active	Exercise 6-7 Days/Week + Physical Job/2x Training
I Want my Weight to	
Decrease	

Goal Start Date	Goal Target Date
....../...../2........	....../...../2........

Date	Week Day	Weight	BMR	Cal Consumed
....	....	....	....	....
....	....	....	....	....
....	....	....	....	....
....	....	....	....	....
....	....	....	....	....
....	....	....	....	....
....	....	....	....	....

It's not recommended that you decrease your calorie intake by more than 1000 calories below your daily calorie needs or consume less than 1800 calories per day.

Goal target date is based on the recommended average weight loss of .45 kg per week.

Measurement System	Current Weight	Age	
Height in m	Centimeters	Goal Weight	Gender
Initial Daily Calorie Needs	Initial Daily Calorie Intake	Calories to Burn	

Cal Burned	Cal Deficit	Cal Remaining	Kgs Remaining	Loss	% of Goal

CALORIES AMORTIZATION SCHEDULE

Extra Active	Exercise 6-7 Days/Week + Physical Job/2x Training			
I Want my Weight to				
Decrease				

Goal Start Date ....../...../2........			Goal Target Date ....../...../2........		

Date	Week Day		Weight	BMR	Cal Consumed
....		....	....	....	....
....		....	....	....	....
....		....	....	....	....
....		....	....	....	....
....		....	....	....	....
....		....	....	....	....
....		....	....	....	....

It's not recommended that you decrease your calorie intake by more than 1000 calories below your daily calorie needs or consume less than 1800 calories per day.

Goal target date is based on the recommended average weight loss of .45 kg per week.

Measurement System		Current Weight		Age	
Height in m	Centimeters	Goal Weight		Gender	
Initial Daily Calorie Needs		Initial Daily Calorie Intake		Calories to Burn	
Cal Burned	Cal Deficit	Cal Remaining	Kgs Remaining	Loss	% of Goal

CALORIES AMORTIZATION SCHEDULE

Extra Active	Exercise 6-7 Days/Week + Physical Job/2x Training
I Want my Weight to	
Decrease	

Goal Start Date	Goal Target Date
....../...../2........	....../...../2........

Date	Week Day	Weight	BMR	Cal Consumed
....	....	....	....	....
....	....	....	....	....
....	....	....	....	....
....	....	....	....	....
....	....	....	....	....
....	....	....	....	....
....	....	....	....	....

It's not recommended that you decrease your calorie intake by more than 1000 calories below your daily calorie needs or consume less than 1800 calories per day.

Goal target date is based on the recommended average weight loss of .45 kg per week.

Measurement System	Current Weight		Age	
Height in m	Centimeters	Goal Weight		Gender
Initial Daily Calorie Needs	Initial Daily Calorie Intake		Calories to Burn	

Cal Burned	Cal Deficit	Cal Remaining	Kgs Remaining	Loss	% of Goal

CALORIES AMORTIZATION SCHEDULE

Extra Active	Exercise 6-7 Days/Week + Physical Job/2x Training
I Want my Weight to	
Decrease	

Goal Start Date ....../...../2........			Goal Target Date ....../...../2........		
Date	Week Day		Weight	BMR	Cal Consumed
....		....	....	....	....
....		....	....	....	....
....		....	....	....	....
....		....	....	....	....
....		....	....	....	....
....		....	....	....	....
....		....	....	....	....

It's not recommended that you decrease your calorie intake by more than 1000 calories below your daily calorie needs or consume less than 1800 calories per day.

Goal target date is based on the recommended average weight loss of .45 kg per week.

Measurement System		Current Weight		Age	
Height in m	Centimeters	Goal Weight		Gender	
Initial Daily Calorie Needs		Initial Daily Calorie Intake		Calories to Burn	

Cal Burned	Cal Deficit	Cal Remaining	Kgs Remaining	Loss	% of Goal

CALORIES AMORTIZATION SCHEDULE

Extra Active	Exercise 6-7 Days/Week + Physical Job/2x Training
I Want my Weight to	
Decrease	

Goal Start Date			Goal Target Date		
....../...../2........			....../...../2........		

Date	Week Day		Weight	BMR	Cal Consumed
....		....	....	....	....
....		....	....	....	....
....		....	....	....	....
....		....	....	....	....
....		....	....	....	....
....		....	....	....	....
....		....	....	....	....

It's not recommended that you decrease your calorie intake by more than 1000 calories below your daily calorie needs or consume less than 1800 calories per day.

Goal target date is based on the recommended average weight loss of .45 kg per week.

Measurement System		Current Weight		Age	
Height in m	Centimeters	Goal Weight		Gender	
Initial Daily Calorie Needs		Initial Daily Calorie Intake		Calories to Burn	
Cal Burned	Cal Deficit	Cal Remaining	Kgs Remaining	Loss	% of Goal

CALORIES AMORTIZATION SCHEDULE

Extra Active	Exercise 6-7 Days/Week + Physical Job/2x Training
I Want my Weight to	
Decrease	

Goal Start Date		Goal Target Date		
....../...../2........		....../...../2........		

Date	Week Day	Weight	BMR	Cal Consumed
....	....	....	....	....
....	....	....	....	....
....	....	....	....	....
....	....	....	....	....
....	....	....	....	....
....	....	....	....	....
....	....	....	....	....

It's not recommended that you decrease your calorie intake by more than 1000 calories below your daily calorie needs or consume less than 1800 calories per day.

Goal target date is based on the recommended average weight loss of .45 kg per week.

Measurement System		Current Weight		Age	
Height in m	Centimeters	Goal Weight		Gender	
Initial Daily Calorie Needs		Initial Daily Calorie Intake		Calories to Burn	
Cal Burned	Cal Deficit	Cal Remaining	Kgs Remaining	Loss	% of Goal

CALORIES AMORTIZATION SCHEDULE

Extra Active	Exercise 6-7 Days/Week + Physical Job/2x Training		
I Want my Weight to			
Decrease			

Goal Start Date		Goal Target Date		
....../...../2........		....../...../2........		

Date	Week Day	Weight	BMR	Cal Consumed
....	....	....	....	....
....	....	....	....	....
....	....	....	....	....
....	....	....	....	....
....	....	....	....	....
....	....	....	....	....
....	....	....	....	....

It's not recommended that you decrease your calorie intake by more than 1000 calories below your daily calorie needs or consume less than 1800 calories per day.

Goal target date is based on the recommended average weight loss of .45 kg per week.

Measurement System		Current Weight		Age	
Height in m	Centimeters	Goal Weight		Gender	
Initial Daily Calorie Needs		Initial Daily Calorie Intake		Calories to Burn	
Cal Burned	Cal Deficit	Cal Remaining	Kgs Remaining	Loss	% of Goal

CALORIES AMORTIZATION SCHEDULE

Extra Active	Exercise 6-7 Days/Week + Physical Job/2x Training
I Want my Weight to	
Decrease	

Goal Start Date			Goal Target Date		
....../...../2........			....../...../2........		

Date	Week Day	Weight	BMR	Cal Consumed
....	....	....	....	....
....	....	....	....	....
....	....	....	....	....
....	....	....	....	....
....	....	....	....	....
....	....	....	....	....
....	....	....	....	....

It's not recommended that you decrease your calorie intake by more than 1000 calories below your daily calorie needs or consume less than 1800 calories per day.

Goal target date is based on the recommended average weight loss of .45 kg per week.

Measurement System		Current Weight		Age	
Height in m	Centimeters	Goal Weight		Gender	
Initial Daily Calorie Needs		Initial Daily Calorie Intake		Calories to Burn	
Cal Burned	Cal Deficit	Cal Remaining	Kgs Remaining	Loss	% of Goal

CALORIES AMORTIZATION SCHEDULE

Extra Active	Exercise 6-7 Days/Week + Physical Job/2x Training
I Want my Weight to	
Decrease	

Goal Start Date			Goal Target Date		
...../...../2........			....../...../2........		

Date	Week Day		Weight	BMR	Cal Consumed
....		....	....	....	....
....		....	....	....	....
....		....	....	....	....
....		....	....	....	....
....		....	....	....	....
....		....	....	....	....
....		....	....	....	....

It's not recommended that you decrease your calorie intake by more than 1000 calories below your daily calorie needs or consume less than 1800 calories per day.

Goal target date is based on the recommended average weight loss of .45 kg per week.

Measurement System		Current Weight		Age	
Height in m	Centimeters	Goal Weight		Gender	
Initial Daily Calorie Needs		Initial Daily Calorie Intake		Calories to Burn	
Cal Burned	Cal Deficit	Cal Remaining	Kgs Remaining	Loss	% of Goal

CALORIES AMORTIZATION SCHEDULE

Extra Active	Exercise 6-7 Days/Week + Physical Job/2x Training
I Want my Weight to	
Decrease	

Goal Start Date ....../...../2........			Goal Target Date ....../...../2........		
Date	Week Day		Weight	BMR	Cal Consumed
....	....		....	....	....
....	....		....	....	....
....	....		....	....	....
....	....		....	....	....
....	....		....	....	....
....	....		....	....	....
....	....		....	....	....

It's not recommended that you decrease your calorie intake by more than 1000 calories below your daily calorie needs or consume less than 1800 calories per day.

Goal target date is based on the recommended average weight loss of .45 kg per week.

Measurement System		Current Weight		Age	
Height in m	Centimeters	Goal Weight		Gender	
Initial Daily Calorie Needs		Initial Daily Calorie Intake		Calories to Burn	
Cal Burned	Cal Deficit	Cal Remaining	Kgs Remaining	Loss	% of Goal

CALORIES AMORTIZATION SCHEDULE

Extra Active	Exercise 6-7 Days/Week + Physical Job/2x Training
I Want my Weight to	
Decrease	

Goal Start Date ....../...../2........	Goal Target Date ....../...../2........

Date	Week Day	Weight	BMR	Cal Consumed
....	....	....	....	....
....	....	....	....	....
....	....	....	....	....
....	....	....	....	....
....	....	....	....	....
....	....	....	....	....
....	....	....	....	....

It's not recommended that you decrease your calorie intake by more than 1000 calories below your daily calorie needs or consume less than 1800 calories per day.

Goal target date is based on the recommended average weight loss of .45 kg per week.

Measurement System		Current Weight		Age	
Height in m	Centimeters	Goal Weight		Gender	
Initial Daily Calorie Needs		Initial Daily Calorie Intake		Calories to Burn	
Cal Burned	Cal Deficit	Cal Remaining	Kgs Remaining	Loss	% of Goal

CALORIES AMORTIZATION SCHEDULE

Extra Active	Exercise 6-7 Days/Week + Physical Job/2x Training			
I Want my Weight to				
Decrease				

Goal Start Date		Goal Target Date		
....../ ...../2........		....../ ...../2........		

Date	Week Day	Weight	BMR	Cal Consumed
....	....	....	....	....
....	....	....	....	....
....	....	....	....	....
....	....	....	....	....
....	....	....	....	....
....	....	....	....	....
....	....	....	....	....

It's not recommended that you decrease your calorie intake by more than 1000 calories below your daily calorie needs or consume less than 1800 calories per day.

Goal target date is based on the recommended average weight loss of .45 kg per week.

Measurement System		Current Weight		Age	
Height in m	Centimeters	Goal Weight		Gender	
Initial Daily Calorie Needs		Initial Daily Calorie Intake		Calories to Burn	
Cal Burned	Cal Deficit	Cal Remaining	Kgs Remaining	Loss	% of Goal

CALORIES AMORTIZATION SCHEDULE

Extra Active	Exercise 6-7 Days/Week + Physical Job/2x Training
I Want my Weight to	
Decrease	

Goal Start Date	Goal Target Date
....../...../2........	....../...../2........

Date	Week Day	Weight	BMR	Cal Consumed
....	....	....	....	....
....	....	....	....	....
....	....	....	....	....
....	....	....	....	....
....	....	....	....	....
....	....	....	....	....
....	....	....	....	....

It's not recommended that you decrease your calorie intake by more than 1000 calories below your daily calorie needs or consume less than 1800 calories per day.

Goal target date is based on the recommended average weight loss of .45 kg per week.

Measurement System		Current Weight		Age	
Height in m	Centimeters	Goal Weight		Gender	
Initial Daily Calorie Needs		Initial Daily Calorie Intake		Calories to Burn	

Cal Burned	Cal Deficit	Cal Remaining	Kgs Remaining	Loss	% of Goal

CALORIES AMORTIZATION SCHEDULE

Extra Active	Exercise 6-7 Days/Week + Physical Job/2x Training
I Want my Weight to	
Decrease	

| Goal Start Date ....../...../2........ | Goal Target Date ....../...../2........ |

Date	Week Day	Weight	BMR	Cal Consumed
....	....	....	....	....
....	....	....	....	....
....	....	....	....	....
....	....	....	....	....
....	....	....	....	....
....	....	....	....	....
....	....	....	....	....

It's not recommended that you decrease your calorie intake by more than 1000 calories below your daily calorie needs or consume less than 1800 calories per day.

Goal target date is based on the recommended average weight loss of .45 kg per week.

Measurement System		Current Weight		Age	
Height in m	Centimeters	Goal Weight		Gender	
Initial Daily Calorie Needs		Initial Daily Calorie Intake		Calories to Burn	

Cal Burned	Cal Deficit	Cal Remaining	Kgs Remaining	Loss	% of Goal

CALORIES AMORTIZATION SCHEDULE

Extra Active	Exercise 6-7 Days/Week + Physical Job/2x Training
I Want my Weight to	
Decrease	

Goal Start Date	Goal Target Date
....../...../2........	....../...../2........

Date	Week	Day	Weight	BMR	Cal Consumed
....		....	....	....	....
....		....	....	....	....
....		....	....	....	....
....		....	....	....	....
....		....	....	....	....
....		....	....	....	....
....		....	....	....	....

It's not recommended that you decrease your calorie intake by more than 1000 calories below your daily calorie needs or consume less than 1800 calories per day.

Goal target date is based on the recommended average weight loss of .45 kg per week.

Measurement System		Current Weight		Age	
Height in m	Centimeters	Goal Weight		Gender	
Initial Daily Calorie Needs		Initial Daily Calorie Intake		Calories to Burn	
Cal Burned	Cal Deficit	Cal Remaining	Kgs Remaining	Loss	% of Goal

CALORIES AMORTIZATION SCHEDULE

Extra Active	Exercise 6-7 Days/Week + Physical Job/2x Training
I Want my Weight to	
Decrease	

Goal Start Date		Goal Target Date		
....../...../2........		....../...../2........		
Date	Week Day	Weight	BMR	Cal Consumed
....	....	....	....	....
....	....	....	....	....
....	....	....	....	....
....	....	....	....	....
....	....	....	....	....
....	....	....	....	....
....	....	....	....	....

It's not recommended that you decrease your calorie intake by more than 1000 calories below your daily calorie needs or consume less than 1800 calories per day.

Goal target date is based on the recommended average weight loss of .45 kg per week.

Measurement System		Current Weight		Age	
Height in m	Centimeters	Goal Weight		Gender	
Initial Daily Calorie Needs		Initial Daily Calorie Intake		Calories to Burn	
Cal Burned	Cal Deficit	Cal Remaining	Kgs Remaining	Loss	% of Goal

CALORIES AMORTIZATION SCHEDULE

Extra Active	Exercise 6-7 Days/Week + Physical Job/2x Training
I Want my Weight to	
Decrease	

Goal Start Date	Goal Target Date
....../...../2........	....../...../2........

Date	Week Day	Weight	BMR	Cal Consumed
....	....	....	....	....
....	....	....	....	....
....	....	....	....	....
....	....	....	....	....
....	....	....	....	....
....	....	....	....	....
....	....	....	....	....

It's not recommended that you decrease your calorie intake by more than 1000 calories below your daily calorie needs or consume less than 1800 calories per day.

Goal target date is based on the recommended average weight loss of .45 kg per week.

Measurement System		Current Weight		Age	
Height in m	Centimeters	Goal Weight		Gender	
Initial Daily Calorie Needs		Initial Daily Calorie Intake		Calories to Burn	

Cal Burned	Cal Deficit	Cal Remaining	Kgs Remaining	Loss	% of Goal

CALORIES AMORTIZATION SCHEDULE

Extra Active	Exercise 6-7 Days/Week + Physical Job/2x Training			
I Want my Weight to				
Decrease				

Goal Start Date		Goal Target Date		
....../...../2........		....../...../2........		

Date	Week Day	Weight	BMR	Cal Consumed
....	....	....	....	....
....	....	....	....	....
....	....	....	....	....
....	....	....	....	....
....	....	....	....	....
....	....	....	....	....
....	....	....	....	....

It's not recommended that you decrease your calorie intake by more than 1000 calories below your daily calorie needs or consume less than 1800 calories per day.

Goal target date is based on the recommended average weight loss of .45 kg per week.

Measurement System		Current Weight		Age	
Height in m	Centimeters	Goal Weight		Gender	
Initial Daily Calorie Needs		Initial Daily Calorie Intake		Calories to Burn	
Cal Burned	Cal Deficit	Cal Remaining	Kgs Remaining	Loss	% of Goal

CALORIES AMORTIZATION SCHEDULE

Extra Active	Exercise 6-7 Days/Week + Physical Job/2x Training
I Want my Weight to	
Decrease	

Goal Start Date ....../...../2........			Goal Target Date ....../...../2........		
Date	Week Day		Weight	BMR	Cal Consumed
....	....		....	....	....
....	....		....	....	....
....	....		....	....	....
....	....		....	....	....
....	....		....	....	....
....	....		....	....	....
....	....		....	....	....

It's not recommended that you decrease your calorie intake by more than 1000 calories below your daily calorie needs or consume less than 1800 calories per day.

Goal target date is based on the recommended average weight loss of .45 kg per week.

Measurement System	Current Weight		Age	

Height in m	Centimeters	Goal Weight		Gender	

Initial Daily Calorie Needs	Initial Daily Calorie Intake		Calories to Burn	

Cal Burned	Cal Deficit	Cal Remaining	Kgs Remaining	Loss	% of Goal

CALORIES AMORTIZATION SCHEDULE

Extra Active	Exercise 6-7 Days/Week + Physical Job/2x Training
I Want my Weight to	
Decrease	

Goal Start Date ....../...../2........			Goal Target Date ....../...../2........		
Date	Week Day		Weight	BMR	Cal Consumed
....		....	....	....	....
....		....	....	....	....
....		....	....	....	....
....		....	....	....	....
....		....	....	....	....
....		....	....	....	....
....		....	....	....	....

It's not recommended that you decrease your calorie intake by more than 1000 calories below your daily calorie needs or consume less than 1800 calories per day.

Goal target date is based on the recommended average weight loss of .45 kg per week.

Measurement System		Current Weight		Age	
Height in m	Centimeters	Goal Weight		Gender	
Initial Daily Calorie Needs		Initial Daily Calorie Intake		Calories to Burn	
Cal Burned	Cal Deficit	Cal Remaining	Kgs Remaining	Loss	% of Goal

CALORIES AMORTIZATION SCHEDULE

Extra Active	Exercise 6-7 Days/Week + Physical Job/2x Training
I Want my Weight to	
Decrease	

Goal Start Date			Goal Target Date		
....../...../2........			....../...../2........		

Date	Week Day	Weight	BMR	Cal Consumed
....	....	....	....	....
....	....	....	....	....
....	....	....	....	....
....	....	....	....	....
....	....	....	....	....
....	....	....	....	....
....	....	....	....	....

It's not recommended that you decrease your calorie intake by more than 1000 calories below your daily calorie needs or consume less than 1800 calories per day.

Goal target date is based on the recommended average weight loss of .45 kg per week.

Measurement System	Current Weight		Age	
Height in m / Centimeters	Goal Weight		Gender	
Initial Daily Calorie Needs	Initial Daily Calorie Intake		Calories to Burn	

Cal Burned	Cal Deficit	Cal Remaining	Kgs Remaining	Loss	% of Goal

CALORIES AMORTIZATION SCHEDULE

Extra Active	Exercise 6-7 Days/Week + Physical Job/2x Training
I Want my Weight to	
Decrease	

Goal Start Date			Goal Target Date		
....../...../2........			....../...../2........		

Date	Week Day	Weight	BMR	Cal Consumed
....	....	....	....	....
....	....	....	....	....
....	....	....	....	....
....	....	....	....	....
....	....	....	....	....
....	....	....	....	....
....	....	....	....	....

It's not recommended that you decrease your calorie intake by more than 1000 calories below your daily calorie needs or consume less than 1800 calories per day.

Goal target date is based on the recommended average weight loss of .45 kg per week.

Measurement System		Current Weight		Age	
Height in m	Centimeters	Goal Weight		Gender	
Initial Daily Calorie Needs		Initial Daily Calorie Intake		Calories to Burn	
Cal Burned	Cal Deficit	Cal Remaining	Kgs Remaining	Loss	% of Goal

CALORIES AMORTIZATION SCHEDULE

Extra Active	Exercise 6-7 Days/Week + Physical Job/2x Training
I Want my Weight to	
Decrease	

Goal Start Date ....../...../2........			Goal Target Date ....../...../2........		
Date	Week Day		Weight	BMR	Cal Consumed
....		....	....	....	....
....		....	....	....	....
....		....	....	....	....
....		....	....	....	....
....		....	....	....	....
....		....	....	....	....
....		....	....	....	....

It's not recommended that you decrease your calorie intake by more than 1000 calories below your daily calorie needs or consume less than 1800 calories per day.

Goal target date is based on the recommended average weight loss of .45 kg per week.

Measurement System		Current Weight		Age	
Height in m	Centimeters	Goal Weight		Gender	
Initial Daily Calorie Needs		Initial Daily Calorie Intake		Calories to Burn	
Cal Burned	Cal Deficit	Cal Remaining	Kgs Remaining	Loss	% of Goal

CALORIES AMORTIZATION SCHEDULE

Extra Active	Exercise 6-7 Days/Week + Physical Job/2x Training
I Want my Weight to	
Decrease	

Goal Start Date ....../...../2........			Goal Target Date ....../...../2........		
Date	Week Day		Weight	BMR	Cal Consumed
....		....	....	....	....
....		....	....	....	....
....		....	....	....	....
....		....	....	....	....
....		....	....	....	....
....		....	....	....	....
....		....	....	....	....

It's not recommended that you decrease your calorie intake by more than 1000 calories below your daily calorie needs or consume less than 1800 calories per day.

Goal target date is based on the recommended average weight loss of .45 kg per week.

Measurement System		Current Weight		Age	
Height in m	Centimeters	Goal Weight		Gender	
Initial Daily Calorie Needs		Initial Daily Calorie Intake		Calories to Burn	
Cal Burned	Cal Deficit	Cal Remaining	Kgs Remaining	Loss	% of Goal

CALORIES AMORTIZATION SCHEDULE

Extra Active	Exercise 6-7 Days/Week + Physical Job/2x Training
I Want my Weight to	
Decrease	

Goal Start Date ....../...../2........	Goal Target Date ....../...../2........

Date	Week Day	Weight	BMR	Cal Consumed
....	....	....	....	....
....	....	....	....	....
....	....	....	....	....
....	....	....	....	....
....	....	....	....	....
....	....	....	....	....
....	....	....	....	....

It's not recommended that you decrease your calorie intake by more than 1000 calories below your daily calorie needs or consume less than 1800 calories per day.

Goal target date is based on the recommended average weight loss of .45 kg per week.

Measurement System	Current Weight		Age	
Height in m	Centimeters	Goal Weight		Gender
Initial Daily Calorie Needs		Initial Daily Calorie Intake		Calories to Burn

Cal Burned	Cal Deficit	Cal Remaining	Kgs Remaining	Loss	% of Goal

CALORIES AMORTIZATION SCHEDULE

Extra Active	Exercise 6-7 Days/Week + Physical Job/2x Training

I Want my Weight to

Decrease

Goal Start Date	Goal Target Date
...../...../2........	...../...../2........

Date	Week Day	Weight	BMR	Cal Consumed
....	....	....	....	....
....	....	....	....	....
....	....	....	....	....
....	....	....	....	....
....	....	....	....	....
....	....	....	....	....
....	....	....	....	....

It's not recommended that you decrease your calorie intake by more than 1000 calories below your daily calorie needs or consume less than 1800 calories per day.

Goal target date is based on the recommended average weight loss of .45 kg per week.

Measurement System		Current Weight		Age	
Height in m	Centimeters	Goal Weight		Gender	
Initial Daily Calorie Needs		Initial Daily Calorie Intake		Calories to Burn	
Cal Burned	Cal Deficit	Cal Remaining	Kgs Remaining	Loss	% of Goal

CALORIES AMORTIZATION SCHEDULE

Extra Active	Exercise 6-7 Days/Week + Physical Job/2x Training				
I Want my Weight to					
Decrease					
Goal Start Date ....../...../2........		Goal Target Date ....../...../2........			
Date	Week Day		Weight	BMR	Cal Consumed
....	....		....	....	....
....	....		....	....	....
....	....		....	....	....
....	....		....	....	....
....	....		....	....	....
....	....		....	....	....
....	....		....	....	....

It's not recommended that you decrease your calorie intake by more than 1000 calories below your daily calorie needs or consume less than 1800 calories per day.

Goal target date is based on the recommended average weight loss of .45 kg per week.

Measurement System	Current Weight		Age	

Height in m	Centimeters	Goal Weight		Gender	

Initial Daily Calorie Needs	Initial Daily Calorie Intake		Calories to Burn	

Cal Burned	Cal Deficit	Cal Remaining	Kgs Remaining	Loss	% of Goal

CALORIES AMORTIZATION SCHEDULE

Extra Active	Exercise 6-7 Days/Week + Physical Job/2x Training			
I Want my Weight to				
Decrease				
Goal Start Date ....../...../2........		Goal Target Date ....../...../2........		
Date	Week Day	Weight	BMR	Cal Consumed
....	....	....	....	....
....	....	....	....	....
....	....	....	....	....
....	....	....	....	....
....	....	....	....	....
....	....	....	....	....
....	....	....	....	....

It's not recommended that you decrease your calorie intake by more than 1000 calories below your daily calorie needs or consume less than 1800 calories per day.

Goal target date is based on the recommended average weight loss of .45 kg per week.

Measurement System		Current Weight		Age	
Height in m	Centimeters	Goal Weight		Gender	
Initial Daily Calorie Needs		Initial Daily Calorie Intake		Calories to Burn	
Cal Burned	Cal Deficit	Cal Remaining	Kgs Remaining	Loss	% of Goal

CALORIES AMORTIZATION SCHEDULE

Extra Active	Exercise 6-7 Days/Week + Physical Job/2x Training
I Want my Weight to	
Decrease	

Goal Start Date	Goal Target Date
....../...../2........	....../...../2........

Date	Week Day	Weight	BMR	Cal Consumed
....	....	....	....	....
....	....	....	....	....
....	....	....	....	....
....	....	....	....	....
....	....	....	....	....
....	....	....	....	....
....	....	....	....	....

It's not recommended that you decrease your calorie intake by more than 1000 calories below your daily calorie needs or consume less than 1800 calories per day.

Goal target date is based on the recommended average weight loss of .45 kg per week.

Measurement System		Current Weight		Age	
Height in m	Centimeters	Goal Weight		Gender	
Initial Daily Calorie Needs		Initial Daily Calorie Intake		Calories to Burn	
Cal Burned	Cal Deficit	Cal Remaining	Kgs Remaining	Loss	% of Goal

www.ingramcontent.com/pod-product-compliance
Lightning Source LLC
Chambersburg PA
CBHW070434290526
45791CB00005B/1976